Health Psychology Research Focus Series

PAIN CONTROL SUPPORT FOR PEOPLE WITH CANCER

Health Psychology Research Focus Series

Parental Treatment and Mental Health of Personality
Ferenc Margitics and Zsuzsa Pauwlik
2009. ISBN: 978-1-60741-318-9

Pain Control Support for People with Cancer
National Cancer Institute
2009. ISBN: 978-1-60692-848-6

Health Psychology Research Focus Series

PAIN CONTROL SUPPORT FOR PEOPLE WITH CANCER

NATIONAL CANCER INSTITUTE

Nova Biomedical Books
New York

Copyright © 2009 by Nova Science Publishers, Inc.

All rights reserved. No part of this book may be reproduced, stored in a retrieval system or transmitted in any form or by any means: electronic, electrostatic, magnetic, tape, mechanical photocopying, recording or otherwise without the written permission of the Publisher.

For permission to use material from this book please contact us:
Telephone 631-231-7269; Fax 631-231-8175
Web Site: http://www.novapublishers.com

NOTICE TO THE READER

The Publisher has taken reasonable care in the preparation of this book, but makes no expressed or implied warranty of any kind and assumes no responsibility for any errors or omissions. No liability is assumed for incidental or consequential damages in connection with or arising out of information contained in this book. The Publisher shall not be liable for any special, consequential, or exemplary damages resulting, in whole or in part, from the readers' use of, or reliance upon, this material.

Independent verification should be sought for any data, advice or recommendations contained in this book. In addition, no responsibility is assumed by the publisher for any injury and/or damage to persons or property arising from any methods, products, instructions, ideas or otherwise contained in this publication.

This publication is designed to provide accurate and authoritative information with regard to the subject matter covered herein. It is sold with the clear understanding that the Publisher is not engaged in rendering legal or any other professional services. If legal or any other expert assistance is required, the services of a competent person should be sought. FROM A DECLARATION OF PARTICIPANTS JOINTLY ADOPTED BY A COMMITTEE OF THE AMERICAN BAR ASSOCIATION AND A COMMITTEE OF PUBLISHERS.

Library of Congress Cataloging-in-Publication Data

Pain control support for people with cancer / National Cancer Institute.
  p. cm.
 Includes index.
 ISBN 978-1-60692-848-6 (softcover)
 1. Cancer pain--Treatment. I. National Cancer Institute (U.S.)
 RC262.P345 2009
 616.99'4--dc22
                                                        2009029572

Published by Nova Science Publishers, Inc. ✛ *New York*

Contents

Preface vii

Chapter 1   What You Should Know about Treating Cancer Pain   1

Chapter 2   Types and Causes of Cancer Pain   5

Chapter 3   Talking about Your Pain   9

Chapter 4   Your Pain Control Plan   15

Chapter 5   Medicines to Treat Cancer Pain   19

Questions to Ask Your Health Care Team About Your Pain Medicine   31

Chapter 6   Medicine Tolerance and Addiction   33

Chapter 7   Other Ways to Control Pain   37

Chapter 8   Your Feelings and Pain   43

Chapter 9   Financial Issues   47

Reflection   51

Resources   53

Pain Control Record   57

How to Use Imagery   59

Words to Know 63

Before You Go to the Pharmacy—Know What You're Getting! 69

Index 71

Preface*

Having cancer doesn't mean that you'll have pain. But if you do, you can manage most of your pain with medicine and other treatments.

This booklet will show you how to work with your doctors, nurses, and others to find the best way to control your pain. It will discuss causes of pain, medicines, how to talk to your doctor, and other topics that may help you.

Chapter 1 - People who have cancer don't always have pain. Everyone is different. But if you do have cancer pain, you should know that you don't have to accept it. Cancer pain can almost always be relieved.

Chapter 2 - Cancer pain can range from mild to very severe. Some days it can be worse than others. It can be caused by the cancer itself, the treatment, or both.

You may also have pain that has nothing to do with your cancer. Some people have other health issues or headaches and muscle strains. But always check with your doctor before taking any over-the-counter medicine to relieve everyday aches and pains.

Chapter 3 - The most important member of the team is you. You're the only one who knows what your pain feels like. Talking about pain is important. It gives your health care team the feedback they need to make you feel better.

Chapter 4 - Your pain control plan will be designed for you and your body. Everyone has a different pain control plan. Even if you have the same type of cancer as someone else, your plan may be different.

Chapter 5 - Your doctor prescribes medicine based on the kind of pain you have and how severe it is. In studies, these medicines have been shown to help control cancer pain. Doctors use three main groups of drugs for pain: nonopioids, opioids, and other types. You may also hear the term analgesics used for these pain relievers. Some are stronger than others. It helps to know the different kinds of medicines, why and how they're used, how you take them, and what side effects you might expect.

Chapter 6 - Addiction is when people can't control their seeking or craving for something. They continue to do something even when it causes them harm. People with cancer often need strong medicine to help control their pain. Yet some people are so afraid of becoming addicted to pain medicine that they won't take it. Family members may also worry that their loved ones will get addicted to pain medicine. Therefore, they sometimes encourage loved ones to "hold off" between doses But even though they may mean well, it's best to take your medicine as prescribed.

Chapter 7- Along with your pain medicine, your health care team may suggest you try other methods to control your pain. However, unlike pain medicine, some of these methods have not been tested in cancer pain studies. But they may help improve your quality of life by helping you with your pain, as well as stress, anxiety, and coping with cancer. Some of these methods are called complementary or integrative.

Chapter 8 - Having pain and cancer affects every part of your life. It can affect not only your body, but your thoughts and feelings as well. Whether you have a lot of pain or a little, if it's constant, you may feel like you aren't able to focus on anything else. It may keep you from doing things and seeing people that you normally do. This can be upsetting and may feel like a cycle that never seems to end.

Chapter 9 - When you're in pain, the last thing you want to think about is paying for your medicine. Yet money worries have stopped many people from getting the pain treatment they need. Talk with your oncology social worker if you have questions. He or she should be able to direct you to resources in your area.

---

* This is an edited, reformatted and augmented version of a National Institute of Health publication 07-6287, revised January 2008.

Chapter 1

What You Should Know about Treating Cancer Pain

You Don't Have to Accept Pain

People who have cancer don't always have pain. Everyone is different. But if you do have cancer pain, you should know that you don't have to accept it. Cancer pain can almost always be relieved.

The key messages we want you to learn from this booklet are:

- Your pain **can** be managed.
- Controlling pain **is part** of your cancer treatment.
- Talking openly with your doctor and health care team will help them manage your pain.
- The best way to control pain is to stop it from starting or keep it from getting worse.
- There are many different medicines to control pain. Everyone's pain control plan is different.
- Keeping a record of your pain will help create the best pain control plan for you.
- People who take cancer pain medicines as prescribed rarely become addicted to them.
- Your body does **not** become immune to pain medicine. Stronger medicines should not be saved for "later."

Pain Specialists Can Help

Cancer pain can be reduced so that you can enjoy your normal routines and sleep better. It may help to talk with a pain specialist. These may be oncologists, **anesthesiologists, neurologists**, surgeons, other doctors, nurses, or pharmacists. If you have a pain control team, it may also include psychologists and social workers.

Pain and **palliative care** specialists are experts in pain control. Palliative care specialists treat the symptoms, **side effects**, and emotional problems of both cancer and its treatment. They will work with you to find the best way to manage your pain. Ask your doctor or nurse to suggest someone. Or contact one of the following for help finding a pain specialist in your area:

- Cancer center
- Your local hospital or medical center
- Your primary care provider
- People who belong to pain support groups in your area
- The Center to Advance Palliative Care, www.getpalliativecare.org (for lists of providers in each state)

When cancer pain is not treated properly, you may be:

- Tired
- Depressed
- Angry
- Worried
- Lonely
- Stressed

When cancer pain is managed properly, you can:

Enjoy being active
Sleep better
Enjoy family and friends
Improve your appetite
Enjoy sexual intimacy

Prevent depression

Chapter 2

Types and Causes of Cancer Pain

Cancer pain can range from mild to very severe. Some days it can be worse than others. It can be caused by the cancer itself, the treatment, or both.

You may also have pain that has nothing to do with your cancer. Some people have other health issues or headaches and muscle strains. But always check with your doctor before taking any over-the-counter medicine to relieve everyday aches and pains.

Different Types of Pain

Here are the common terms used to describe different types of pain:

- **Acute pain** ranges from mild to severe. It comes on quickly and lasts a short time.
- **Chronic pain** ranges from mild to severe. It either won't go away or comesback often.
- **Breakthrough pain** is an intense rise in pain that occurs suddenly or is feltfor a short time. It can occur by itself or in relation to a certain activity. Itmay happen several times a day, even when you're taking the right dose ofmedicine. For example, it may happen as the current dose of your medicine is wearing off.

What Causes Cancer Pain?

Cancer and its treatment cause most cancer pain. Major causes of pain include:

- **Pain from medical tests.** Some methods used to diagnose cancer or seehow well treatment is working are painful. Examples may be a biopsy, spinaltap, or bone marrow test. If you are told you need the procedure, don't letconcerns about pain stop you from having it done. Talk with your doctorahead of time about what will be done to lessen any pain you may have.
- **Pain from a tumor.** If the cancer grows bigger or spreads, it can cause painby pressing on the tissues around it. For example, a tumor can cause pain if itpresses on bones, nerves, the spinal cord, or body organs.
- **Spinal cord compression.** When a tumor spreads to the spine, it can press on the spinal cord and cause spinal cord compression. The first sign of this is often back or neck pain, or both. Coughing, sneezing, or other motions may make it worse.
- **Pain from treatment. Chemotherapy, radiation therapy**, surgery, and other treatments may cause pain for some people. Some examples of pain from treatment are:

  - **Neuropathic pain.** This is pain that may occur if treatment damages the nerves. The pain is often burning, sharp, or shooting. The cancer itself can also cause this kind of pain.
  - **Phantom pain.** You may still feel pain or other discomfort coming from a body part that has been removed by surgery. Doctors aren't sure why this happens, but it's real.

How much pain you feel depends on different things. These include where the cancer is in your body, what kind of damage it is causing, and how you experience the pain in *your* body. Everyone is different.

Listen to Your Body

If you notice that everyday actions, such as coughing, sneezing, or moving, cause new pain or your pain to get worse, tell your doctors right away. Also let them know if you have unusual rashes or bowel or bladder change.

Chapter 3

Talking about Your Pain

Pain Control is Part of Treatment: Talking Openly is Key

"At first I tried to be brave. Now I realize that the only way to handle my pain is to be open and honest about it with my health care team. It's the only way I can stay on top of it and keep it under control." —Janie

Controlling Pain is a Key Part of Your Overall Cancer Treatment

The most important member of the team is you. You're the only one who knows what your pain feels like. Talking about pain is important. It gives your health care team the feedback they need to make you feel better.

Some people with cancer don't want to talk about their pain. They think that they'll distract their doctors from working on ways to help treat their cancer. Or they worry that they won't be seen as "good" patients. They also worry that they won't be able to afford pain medicine. As a result, people sometimes get so used to living with their pain that they forget what it's like to live without it.

But your health care team needs to know details about your pain and whether it's getting worse. This helps them understand how the cancer and its treatment are affecting your body. And it helps them figure out how to best control the pain.

Try to talk openly about any other medical problems and fears you have. And if money worries are stopping you, be sure to read the Financial Issues section of this book. There may be ways to help you get the medicine you need.

Tell Your Health Care Team If You're:

- Taking any medicine to treat other health problems
- Taking more or less of the pain medicine than prescribed
- Allergic to certain drugs
- Using any over-the-counter medicines, home remedies, or herbal or alternative therapies

This information could affect the pain control plan your doctor suggests for you. If you feel uneasy talking about your pain, bring a family member or friend to speak for you. Or let your loved one take notes and ask questions. Remember, open communication between you, your loved ones, and your health care team will lead to better pain control.

Talking About Your Pain

The first step in getting your pain under control is talking honestly about it. Try to talk with your health care team and your loved ones about what you are feeling. This means telling them:

- Where you have pain
- What it feels like (sharp, dull, throbbing, constant, burning, or shooting)
- How strong your pain is
- How long it lasts
- What lessens your pain or makes it worse
- When it happens (what time of day, what you're doing, and what's going on)
- If it gets in the way of daily activities

Describe and Rate Your Pain

You will be asked to describe and rate your pain. This provides a way to assess your **pain threshold** and measure how well your pain control plan is working.

Your doctor may ask you to describe your pain in a number of ways. A pain scale is the most common way. The scale uses the numbers 0 to 10, where 0 is no pain, and 10 is the worst. You can also use words to describe pain, like pinching, stinging, or aching. Some doctors show their patients a series of faces and ask them to point to the face that best describes how they feel.

No matter how you or your doctor keep track of your pain, make sure that you do it the same way each time. You also need to talk about any new pain you feel.

It may help to keep a record of your pain. See the chart on page 37 for an example. Some people use a pain diary or journal. Others create a list or a computer spreadsheet. Choose the way that works best for you.

Your record could list:

- When you take pain medicine
- Name and dose of the medicine you're taking
- Any side effects you have
- How long the pain medicine works
- Other pain relief methods you use to control your pain
- Any activity that is affected by pain, or makes it better or worse
- Things that you can't do at all because of the pain

Share your record with your health care team. It can help them figure out how helpful your pain medicines are, or if they need to change your pain control plan.

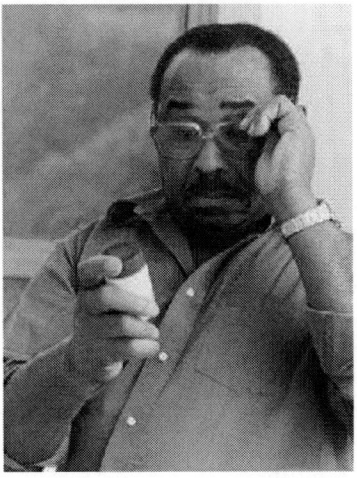

Here Are Some Ways Your Health Care Team May Ask You to Describe or Rate Your Pain

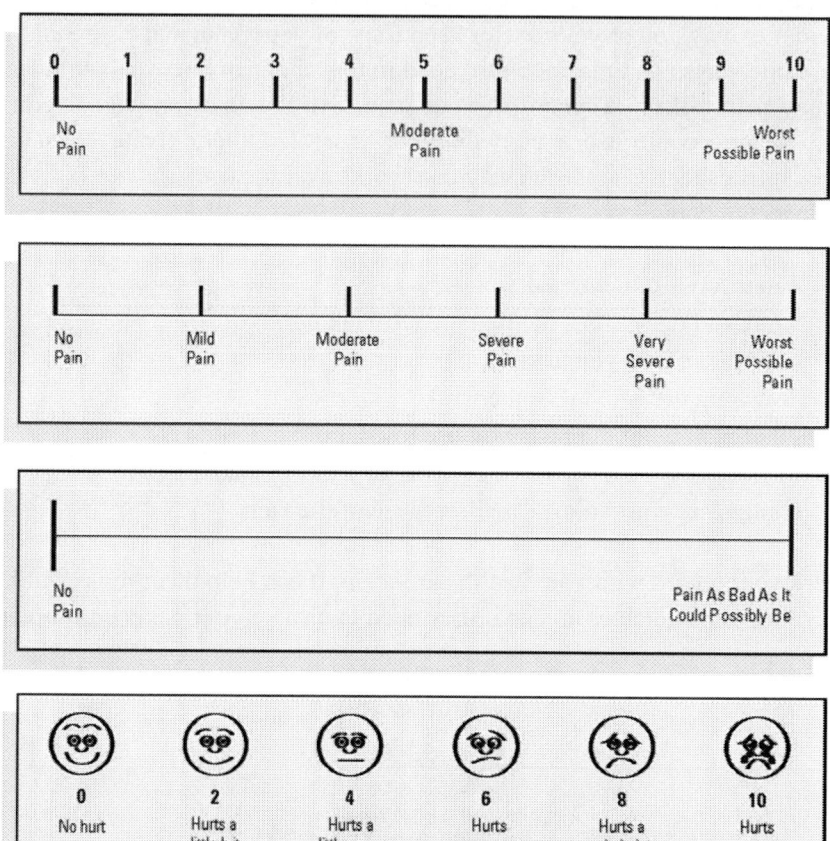

0–10 Numeric Pain Intensity Scale, Simple Descriptive Pain Intensity Scale, and Visual Analog Scale (VAS): Acute Pain Management Guideline Panel. Acute Pain Management in Adults: Operative Procedures. Quick Reference Guide for Clinicians AHCPR Pub. No. 92-0019. Rockville, MD: Agency for Health Care Policy and Research, Public Health Service, U.S. Department of Health and Human Services.

"Faces" Pain Scale adapted with permission from Hockenberry MJ, Wilson D, Winkelstein ML: *Wong's Essentials of Pediatric Nursing*, ed. 7, St. Louis, 2005, p. 1259. Used with permission. Copyright, Mosby.

Share Your Beliefs

Some people don't want to take medicine, even when it's prescribed by the doctor. Taking it may be against religious or cultural beliefs. Or there may be other personal reasons why someone won't take medicine. If you feel any of these ways about pain medicine, it's important to share your views with your health care team. If you prefer, ask a friend or family member to share them for you. Talking openly about your beliefs will help your health care team find a plan that works best for you.

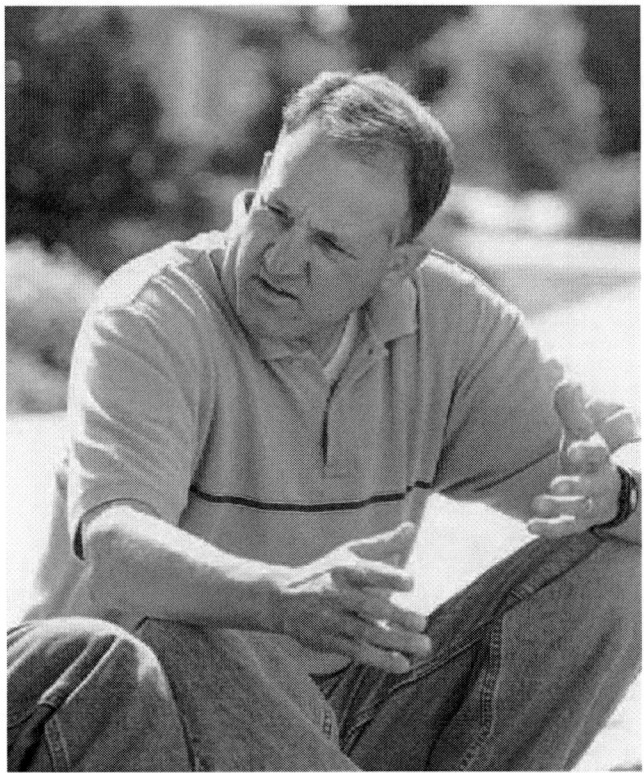

"It makes sense. If you don't tell someone about your pain, then no one can help you! And the pain won't go away by itself." — Joe

Chapter 4

Your Pain Control Plan

"It took a few visits to my health care team to get my pain under control. But by trying different medicines and doses, I now have a pain plan that works for me."

– Michelle

Make Your Pain Control Plan Work for You

Your pain control plan will be designed for you and your body. Everyone has a different pain control plan. Even if you have the same type of cancer as someone else, your plan may be different.

Take your pain medicine **dose** on schedule to keep the pain from starting or getting worse. This is one of the best ways to stay on top of your pain. **Don't skip doses**. Once you feel pain, it's harder to control and may take longer to get better.

Here are some other things you can do:

- Bring your list of medicines to each visit.
- If you are seeing more than one doctor, make sure each one sees your list of medicines, especially if he or she is going to change or prescribe medicine.
- Never take someone else's medicine. What helped a friend or relative may not help you. Do not get medicine from other countries or the Internet without telling your doctor.
- Don't wait for the pain to get worse.
- Ask your doctor to change your pain control plan if it isn't working.

The Best Way to Control Pain is to Stop it before it Starts or Prevent it from Getting Worse

Don't wait until the pain gets bad or unbearable before taking your medicine. Pain is easier to control when it's mild. And you need to take pain medicine often enough to stay ahead of your pain. Follow the dose schedule your doctor gives you. Don't try to "hold off" between doses. If you wait:

- Your pain could get worse.
- It may take longer for the pain to get better or go away.
- You may need larger doses to bring the pain under control.

Keep A List Of All Your Medicines

Make a list of all the medicines you are taking. If you need to, ask a member of your family or health care team to help you. **Bring this list of medicines to each visit.** You can take most pain medicines with other **prescription** drugs. But your health care team needs to know what you take and when. Tell them each drug you are taking, no matter how harmless you think it might be. Even over-the-counter medicines, herbs, and **supplements** can interfere with cancer treatment.

How To Tell When You Need A New Pain Control Plan

Here are a few things to watch out for and tell your health care team about:

- Your pain isn't getting better or going away.
- Your pain medicine doesn't work as fast as your doctor said it would.
- Your pain medicine doesn't work as long as your doctor said it would.
- You have breakthrough pain.
- You have side effects that don't go away.

If you have trouble breathing, dizziness, or rashes, call your doctor right away. You may be having an allergic reaction to the pain medicine.

Don't Give Up Hope. Your Pain *can be* Managed

If you are still having pain that is hard to control, you may want to talk with your health care team about seeing a pain or palliative care specialist (see page 2). Whatever you do, don't give up. If one medicine doesn't work, there is almost always another one to try. Also, new medicines are created all the time. And unlike other medicines, there is no "right" dose for many pain medicines. Your dose may be more or less than someone else's. The right dose is the one that relieves your pain and makes you feel better.

Chapter 5

Medicines to Treat Cancer Pain

There is More Than One Way to Treat Pain

Your doctor prescribes medicine based on the kind of pain you have and how severe it is. In studies, these medicines have been shown to help control cancer pain. **Doctors use three main groups of drugs for pain: nonopioids, opioids**, and other types. You may also hear the term **analgesics** used for these pain relievers. Some are stronger than others. It helps to know the different kinds of medicines, why and how they're used, how you take them, and what side effects you might expect.

1. Nonopioids—For Mild to Moderate Pain

Nonopioids are drugs used to treat mild to moderate pain, fever, and swelling. On a scale of 0 to 10, a nonopioid may be used if you rate your pain from 1 to 4. These medicines are stronger than most people realize. In many cases, they are all you'll need to relieve your pain. You just need to be sure to take them regularly.

You can buy most nonopioids without a prescription. **But you still need to talk with your doctor before taking them.** Some of them may have things added to them that you need to know about. And they do have side effects. Common ones, such as nausea, itching, or drowsiness, usually go away after a few days. **Do not** take more than the label says unless your doctor tells you to do so.

Nonopioids include:

- Acetaminophen, which you may know as Tylenol®
  Acetaminophen reduces pain. It is not helpful with inflammation. Most of the time, people don't have side effects from a normal dose of acetaminophen. But taking largedoses of this medicine every day for a long time can damage your liver. Drinking alcohol with the typical dose can also damage the liver.
  Make sure you tell the doctor that you're taking acetaminophen. Sometimes it is used in other pain medicines, so you may not realize that you're taking morethan you should. Also, your doctor may not want you to take acetaminophen too often if you're getting chemotherapy. The medicine can cover up a fever, hiding the fact that you might have an infection.
- Nonsteroidal anti-inflammatory drugs (NSAIDs), such as ibuprofen (which you may know as Advil® or Motrin®) and aspirin
  NSAIDs help control pain and inflammation. With NSAIDs, the most commonside effect is stomach upset or indigestion, especially in older people. Eating foodor drinking milk when you take these drugs may stop this from happening.

NSAIDs may also keep blood from clotting the way it should. This means that it's harder to stop bleeding after you've hurt yourself. NSAIDs can also sometimes cause bleeding in the stomach.

Tell your doctor if:

- Your stools become darker than normal
- You notice bleeding from your rectum
- You have an upset stomach
- You have heartburn symptoms
- You cough up blood

Acetaminophen and NSAIDs at a Glance

Type	Other Names	Action	Side Effects
Acetaminophen	Tylenol®	Reduces pain and fever	Large doses can damage the liver. May cause liver damage if you drink three or more alcoholic drinks a day. Lowers fever. Talk to your doctor if your body temperature is above normal (98.6°) and you are taking this medicine.
NSAIDs (aspirin, ibuprofen, naproxen)	Bayer® (aspirin) Ecotrin® (aspirin) Advil® (ibuprofen) Motrin® (ibuprofen) Nuprin® (ibuprofen) Aleve® (naproxen)	Reduces pain, inflammation (swelling), and fever	Can upset the stomach. Can cause bleeding of the stomach lining, especially if you drink alcohol (wine, beer, etc.). Can cause kidney problems, especially in the elderly or those with existing kidney problems. Can cause heart problems, especially in those who already have heart disease. However, aspirin does not cause heart problems. Avoid these medicines if you are on anticancer drugs that may cause bleeding. Lowers fever. Talk to your doctor if your body temperature is above normal (98.6°) and you are taking this medicine.

What to Avoid When Taking NSAIDS

Some people have conditions that NSAIDs can make worse. In general, you should avoid these drugs if you:

- Are allergic to aspirin
- Are getting chemotherapy
- Are on **steroid** medicines
- Have stomach ulcers or a history of ulcers, gout, or bleeding disorders
- Are taking prescription medicines for arthritis
- Have kidney problems
- Have heart problems
- Are planning surgery within a week
- Are taking blood-thinning medicine (such as Coumadin®)

2. Opioids—For Moderate to Severe Pain

If you're having moderate to severe pain, your doctor may recommend that you take stronger drugs called opioids. Opioids are also known as narcotics. You must have a doctor's prescription to take them. They are often taken with aspirin, ibuprofen, and acetaminophen.

Common opioids include:

- Codeine
- Methadone
- Fentanyl
  Morphine
- Hydromorphone
- Oxycodone
- Levorphanol
- Oxymorphone
- Meperidine

Getting Relief with Opioids

Over time, people who take opioids for pain sometimes find that they need to take larger doses to get relief. This is caused by more pain, the cancer getting worse, or medicine **tolerance** (see pages 20 and 21). When a medicine doesn't give you enough pain relief, your doctor may increase the dose and how often you take it. He or she can also prescribe a stronger drug. Both methods are safe and effective under your doctor's care. **Do not increase the dose of medicine on your own.**

Managing and Preventing Side Effects

Some pain medicines may cause:

- Constipation (trouble passing stools)
- Drowsiness (feeling sleepy)
- Nausea (upset stomach)
- Vomiting (throwing up)

Usually these side effects last only a few days. But if they last longer, your doctors can change the medicine or dose you're taking. Or they may also add another medicine to your pain control plan to control the side effects. Keep in mind that constipation will only go away if it's treated. Your health care team can talk with you about other ways to relieve side effects. Don't let side effects stop you from getting your pain under control.

Other less common side effects include:

- Dizziness
- Confusion
- Breathing problems
- Itching
- Trouble urinating

Constipation

Almost everyone taking opioids has some constipation. This happens because opioids cause the stool to move more slowly through your system, so your body takes more time to absorb water from the stool. The stool then becomes hard.

You can control or prevent constipation by taking these steps:

- Ask your doctor about giving you **laxatives** and stool **softener's** when you first start taking opioids. Taking these right when you start taking pain medicine may prevent the problem.
- Drink plenty of liquids. Drinking 8 to 10 glasses of liquid each day will help keep stools soft.
- Eat foods high in fiber, including raw fruits with the skin left on, vegetables, and whole grain breads and cereals.
- Add 1 to 2 tablespoons of bran to your food or sprinkle it on your food. Remember to drink a glass of water when you eat bran, or it will make the problem worse.
- Exercise as much as you are able. Any movement, such as light walking, will help.
- Call your doctor if you have not had a bowel movement in 2 days or more.

Drowsiness

If your pain has kept you from sleeping, you may sleep more at first when you begin taking opioids. The drowsiness usually goes away after a few days.

If you are tired or drowsy:

- Don't walk up and down stairs alone.
- Don't do anything where you need to be alert—driving, using machines or equipment, or anything else that requires focus.

Call your doctor if the drowsiness is severe or doesn't go away after a week.

- You may have to take a smaller dose more often or change medicines.
- It may be that the medicine isn't relieving your pain, and the pain is keeping you awake at night.
- Your other medicines may be causing the drowsiness.
- Your doctor may decide to add a new drug that will help you stay awake.

Nausea and Vomiting

Nausea and vomiting usually go away after a few days of taking opioids. These tips may help:

- Stay in bed for an hour or so after taking your medicine if you feel sick when walking around. This kind of nausea is like feeling seasick. Some over-the-counter drugs may help, too. But be sure to check with your doctor before taking any other medicines.
- You may want to ask your doctor to prescribe antinausea drugs.
- Ask your doctor if something else could be making you feel sick. It might be related to your cancer or another medicine you're taking. Constipation can also add to nausea.

Starting A New Pain Medicine

Some pain medicines can make you feel sleepy when you first take them. This usually goes away within a few days. Also, some people get dizzy or feel confused. Tell your doctor if any of these symptoms persist. Changing your dose or the type of medicine can usually solve the problem.

What to Watch Out for When Taking Pain Medicine

All drugs must be taken carefully. Here are a few things to remember when you are taking opioids:

- **Take your medicines as directed.** Also, don't split, chew, or crush them, unless suggested by your doctor.
- **Doctors will adjust the pain medicine dose so that you get the right amount for your body.** That's why it's important that only one doctor prescribes your opioids. Make sure that you bring your list of medicines to each visit. That way, your health care team is aware of your pain control plan.
- **Combining pain medicine with alcohol or tranquilizers can be dangerous.** You could have trouble breathing or feel confused, anxious, or dizzy.

Tell your doctor <u>how much</u> and <u>how often</u> you:

- Drink alcohol
- Take tranquilizers, sleeping pills, or **antidepressants**

- Take any other medicines that make you sleepy

How to Stop Taking Opioids

You may be able to take less medicine when the pain gets better. You may even be able to stop taking opioids. But it's important to stop taking opioids slowly, with your doctor's advice. When pain medicines are taken for long periods of time, your body gets used to them. If the medicines are stopped or suddenly reduced, a condition called **withdrawal** may occur. This is why the doses should be lowered slowly. This has *no* relation to being addicted (see Chapter 6).

Stopping your pain medicines slowly makes withdrawal symptoms mild. But if you stop taking opioids suddenly, you may start feeling like you have the flu. You may sweat and have diarrhea or other symptoms. If this happens, tell your doctor or nurse. He or she can treat these symptoms. Any symptoms from withdrawal may take a few days to a few weeks to go away.

---

3. Other Types of Pain Medicine

Doctors also prescribe other types of medicine to relieve cancer pain. They can be used along with nonopioids and opioids. Some include:

- **Antidepressants.** Some drugs can be used for more than one purpose. Forexample, antidepressants are used to treat depression, but they may also helprelieve tingling and burning pain. Nerve damage from radiation, surgery, orchemotherapy can cause this type of pain.
- **Antiseizure medicines (anticonvulsants).** Like antidepressants, anticonvulsants or antiseizure drugs can also be used to help control tinglingor burning from nerve injury.
- **Steroids.** Steroids are mainly used to treat pain caused by swelling.

Be sure to ask your health care team about the common side effects of these medicines.

How Medicine is Given

To relieve cancer pain, doctors often prescribe pills or liquids. But there are also other ways to take medicines, such as:

- **Mouth:** Some pain medicine can be put inside the cheek or under the tongue.

- **Injections (shots):** There are two different kinds of shots:

    - **Under the skin:** Medicine is placed just under the skin using a small needle. These are called **subcutaneous** injections.
    - **In the vein:** Medicine goes directly into the vein through a needle. These are called **intravenous (IV)** injections. **Patient-controlled analgesia (PCA)** pumps are often used with these kinds of injections. PCA pumps let you push a button to give yourself a dose of pain medicine.

- **Skin patches:** These bandage-like patches go on the skin. They slowly but steadily, release medicine for 2 to 3 days.
- **Rectal suppositories:** These are capsules or pills that you put inside your rectum. The medicine dissolves and is absorbed by the body.
- **Around the spinal cord:** Medicine is placed between the wall of the spinal canal and the covering of the spinal cord (called an **epidural**).

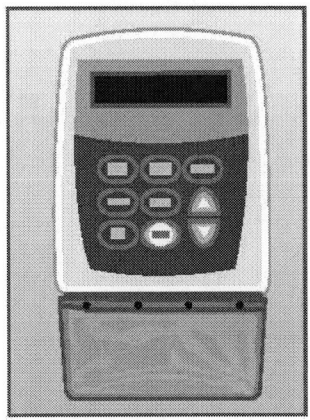

Patient-controlled analgesia pump (PCA)

Questions to Ask Your Health Care Team about Your Pain Medicine

- How much medicine should I take?

  How often?

- If my pain doesn't go away, can I take more medicine?

  How much should I increase the dose?

- Should I call you before taking more medicine?

- How long does the medicine last?

- What if I forget to take my medicine or take it later than I was supposed to?

- Should I take my medicine with food?

- How much liquid should I drink with the medicine?

- How long does it take for the medicine to start working?

- Is it safe to drink alcohol (wine, beer, etc.), drive, or run machinery after I've taken the medicine?

- What other medicines can I take with the pain medicine?

- What are the side effects? How can I prevent them?

- What should I call you about right away?

Other Ways to Relieve Pain

Medicine doesn't always relieve pain in some people. In these cases, doctors use other treatments to reduce pain:

- **Radiation therapy.** Different forms of radiation energy are used to shrink the tumor and reduce pain. Often one treatment is enough to help with the pain. But sometimes several treatments are needed.
- **Neurosurgery.** A surgeon cuts the nerves that carry pain messages to your brain.
- **Nerve blocks.** Anesthesiologists inject pain medicine into or around the nerve or into the spine to relieve pain.
- **Surgery.** A surgeon removes all or part of a tumor to relieve pain. This is especially helpful when a tumor presses on nerves or other parts of the body.

- **Chemotherapy.** Anticancer drugs are used to reduce the size of a tumor, which may help with the pain.
- **Transcutaneous Electric Nerve Stimulation (TENS).** TENS uses a gentle electric current to relieve pain. The current comes from a small power pack that you can hold or attach to yourself.

Questions to Ask Your Health Care Team about Your Pain Medicine

Chapter 6

Medicine Tolerance and Addiction

When Treating Cancer Pain, Addiction is Rarely a Problem

Addiction is when people can't control their seeking or craving for something. They continue to do something even when it causes them harm. People with cancer often need strong medicine to help control their pain. Yet some people are so afraid of becoming addicted to pain medicine that they won't take it. Family members may also worry that their loved ones will get addicted to pain medicine. Therefore, they sometimes encourage loved ones to "hold off" between doses But even though they may mean well, it's best to take your medicine as prescribed.

People in pain get the most relief when they take their medicines on schedule. And don't be afraid to ask for larger doses if you need them. As mentioned on page 13, developing a tolerance to pain medicine is common. But taking cancer pain medicine is not likely to cause addiction. If you're not a drug addict, you won't become one. Even if you have had an addiction problem before, you still deserve good pain management. Talk with your doctor or nurse about your concerns.

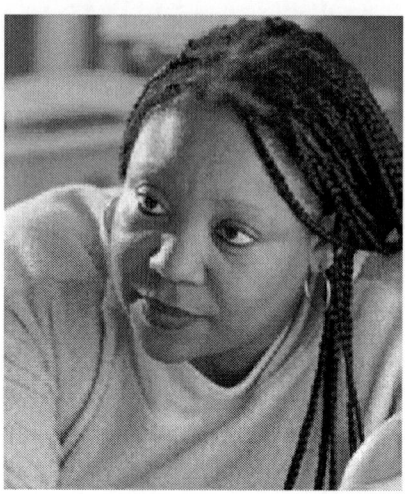

"If you're worried about addiction, ask yourself one question. If you didn't have this pain, would you want this medicine? The answer is usually no." —Robin

Tolerance to Pain Medicine Sometimes Happens

Some people think that they have to save stronger medicines for later. They're afraid that their bodies will get used to the medicine and that it won't work anymore. But medicine doesn't stop working—it just doesn't work as well as it once did. As you keep taking a medicine over time, you may need a change in your pain control plan to get the same amount of relief.

This is called tolerance. Tolerance is a common issue in cancer pain treatment.

Medicine Tolerance is not the Same as Addiction

As mentioned, medicine tolerance happens when your body gets used to the medicine you're taking. Each person's body is different. Many people don't develop a tolerance to opioids. But if tolerance happens to you, don't worry.

Under your doctor's care, you can:

- Increase your dose in small amounts
- Add a new kind of medicine
- Change the kind of medicine that you're taking for pain

The goal is to relieve your pain. Increasing the dose to overcome tolerance does not lead to addiction.

Taking Pain Medicine Will Not Cause You to "Get High"

Most people do not "get high" or lose control when they take cancer pain medicines as prescribed by the doctor. Some pain medicines can cause you to feel sleepy when you first take them This feeling usually goes away within a few days. On occasion, people get dizzy or feel confused when they take pain medicines. Tell your doctor or nurse if this happens to you. Changing your dose or type of medicine can usually solve this problem.

Chapter 7

Other Ways to Control Pain

Along with your pain medicine, your health care team may suggest you try other methods to control your pain. However, unlike pain medicine, some of these methods have not been tested in cancer pain studies. But they may help improve your quality of life by helping you with your pain, as well as stress, anxiety, and coping with cancer. Some of these methods are called complementary or integrative.

These treatments include everything from cold packs, massage, acupuncture, hypnosis, and imagery to biofeedback, meditation, and therapeutic touch. Once you learn how, you can do some of them by yourself. For others, you may have to see a specialist to receive these treatments. If you do, ask if they are licensed experts.

Acupuncture

Acupuncture is a form of Chinese medicine. It involves inserting very thin, metal needles into the skin at certain points of the body. *(Applying pressure to these points with just the thumbs or fingertips is called acupressure.)* The goal is to change the body's energy flow so it can heal itself.

When receiving this treatment, you may have a slight ache, dull pain, tingling, or electrical-feeling sensation for a few seconds after the needles are inserted. Once the needles are in place, though, you shouldn't feel any discomfort. They remain in place for 15 to 30 minutes. However, it may be more or less, depending on what the practitioner suggests.

Acupuncture has been shown to help with nausea and vomiting related to cancer treatment. And some studies have shown it may help with cancer pain. Before getting acupuncture, talk with your health care team to make sure it's safe for your type of cancer. If it is, your health care team can suggest a licensed acupuncturist. Many hospitals and cancer centers have one on staff.

Biofeedback

Biofeedback uses machines to teach you how to control certain body functions, such as heart rate, breathing, and muscle tension. You probably never think of these body functions because they happen on their own. But learning how to control them may help you relax and cope with pain. Biofeedback is often used with other pain relief methods. If you're interested in trying this method, you must see a licensed biofeedback technician.

Distraction

Distraction is simply turning your focus to something other than the pain. It may be used alone to manage mild pain, or used with medicines to help with acute pain, such as pain related to procedures or tests. Or you may try it while waiting for your pain medicine to start working.

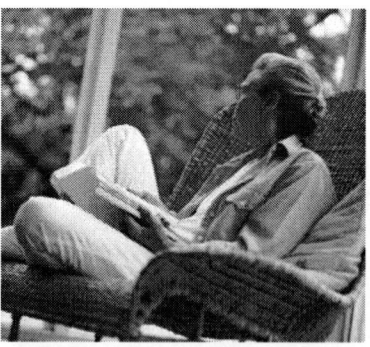

More than likely, you've done this method without realizing it. For example, watching television and listening to music are good ways to distract your mind. In fact, any activity that can focus your attention can be used for distraction. You can count, sing, or pray. You could try slow rhythmic breathing or repeat certain phrases over and over again, such as "I can cope."

You could do certain activities that take your mind from the pain. Some of these may be crafts or hobbies, reading, going to a movie, or visiting friends.

Heat and Cold

Heat may relieve sore muscles, while cold may numb the pain. However, ask your doctor if it is safe to use either during treatment. *Do not* use them for more than 10 minutes at a time. And *do not* use heat or cold over any area where circulation is poor.

For cold, try plastic gel packs that remain soft even when frozen. You can find them in drug and medical-supply stores. Of course, you always can use ice cubes wrapped in a towel or frozen water in a paper cup.

For heat, you can use a heating pad. But you also can try gel packs heated in hot water, hot-water bottles, a hot, moist towel, and hot baths and showers. Be careful not to leave heat on too long to avoid burns.

Hypnosis

Hypnosis is a trance-like state of relaxed and focused attention. People describe it as a lot like the way they feel when they first wake up in the morning. Their eyes are closed, but they're aware of what's going on around them. In this relaxed state, people's minds are usually more receptive or open to suggestion. As a result, hypnosis can be used to block the awareness of pain or to help you change the sensation of pain to a more pleasant one.

You'll need to see a person who is trained in hypnosis, often a psychologist or psychiatrist. He or she may also be able to teach you how to place yourself in a trance-like state, by making positive suggestions to yourself.

Imagery

Imagery is like a daydream. You close your eyes and create images in your mind to help you relax, feel less anxious, and sleep. You daydream using all of your senses – sight, touch, hearing, smell, and taste. For example, you may want to think of a place or activity that made you happy in the past. You could explore this scene, which could help reduce your pain both during and after you try it.

If you have to stay in bed or can't leave the house, imagery may help. It may lessen the closed-in feelings you have after being indoors for a long time. See page 39 for an exercise on how to use imagery.

Massage

Massage may help reduce pain and anxiety. It may also help with fatigue and stress. It is pressing, rubbing, and kneading parts of the body with hands or special tools. For pain, a steady, circular motion near the pain site may work best. Massage may also help relieve tension and increase blood flow. Deep or intense pressure should *not* be used with cancer patients unless their healthcare team says it's okay to do so.

Meditation

Meditation is a form of mind-body medicine used to help relax the body and quiet the mind. It may help with pain, as well as with worry, stress, or depression.

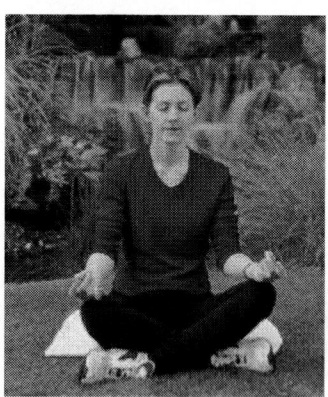

"I began meditating as a way to help relieve my pain and calm myself. I can't avoid medicine, but I feel like I don't have to take as much." —Anna

People who are meditating use certain techniques such as focusing attention on something, like a word or phrase, an object, or the breath. They may sit, lie down, walk, or be in any other position that makes them feel comfortable. A goal while meditating is to try to have an open attitude toward distracting thoughts or emotions. When they occur, attention is gently brought back to breathing or the silent repeating of phrases.

Relaxation

Relaxation reduces pain or keeps it from getting worse by getting rid of tension in your muscles. It may help you sleep and give you more energy. Relaxation may also reduce anxiety and help you cope with stress.

The most common methods of relaxation are:

- **Visual concentration.** When you stare at an object.
- **Breathing and muscle tensing.** This is breathing in and tensing themuscles, then breathing out while letting your muscles go. See page 40 for an exercise on how to use breathing and muscle tensing.
- **Slow rhythmic breathing.** To do this, you breathe slowly in and out whileconcentrating on an object. You can add imagery to slow rhythmic breathingor listen to music too. See page 40 for an exercise on how to use slowrhythmic breathing.

Sometimes, relaxation is hard if you're in severe pain. You could try using some of the methods that are quick and easy. These may be rhythmic massage or breathing and muscle tensing. Some people use music or other types of art therapy to help them relax.

Sometimes breathing too deeply can cause shortness of breath. If this happens, take shallow breaths or breathe more slowly. Also, as you start to relax, you may fall asleep. If you don't want to sleep, sit in a hard chair or set a timer or alarm before you start the exercise.

Other Methods

Here are some other ways people have tried to find relief from cancer pain.

- **Physical Therapy.** Exercises or methods used to help restore strength,increase movement to muscles, and relieve pain.

- **Reiki.** A form of energy medicine in which the provider places his or herhands on or near the patient. The intent is to transmit what is believed to bea life force energy called qi (or chi).
- **Tai Chi.** A mind-body practice that is a series of slow, gentle movementswith a focus on breathing and concentration. The thought is that it helpswhat is believed to be a life force energy (called **qi**) flow through the body.
- **Yoga.** Systems of stretches and poses with special focus given to breathing. It is meant to calm the nervous system and balance the body, mind, and spirit. There are different types of yoga, so ask about which ones would be best for you.

Make sure that you see a licensed expert when trying physical therapy, massage, hypnosis, or acupuncture.

To Learn More about Complementary Treatments for Pain

- Talk with your doctor, nurse, or oncology social worker.
- See the NCI booklet Thinking About Complementary & Alternative Medicine: A Guide for People With Cancer. See page 34 on how to order.
- Contact the National Center for Complementary and Alternative Medicine at 1-888-644-6226 or online at http://nccam.nih.gov.
- See the web site for the NCI Office of Cancer Complementary and Alternative Medicine at www.cancer.gov/cam.

Remember: Always talk with your doctor before using any complementary pain treatments. Some may interfere with your cancer treatment.

Chapter 8

Your Feelings and Pain

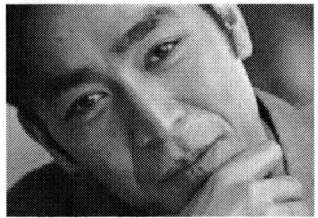

"At first I wasn't able to do the things I used to do. I couldn't mow my lawn or work in my garden. It was very frustrating." —Juan

Having pain and cancer affects every part of your life. It can affect not only your body, but your thoughts and feelings as well. Whether you have a lot of pain or a little, if it's constant, you may feel like you aren't able to focus on anything else. It may keep you from doing things and seeing people that you normally do. This can be upsetting and may feel like a cycle that never seems to end.

Sometimes things that people used to take for granted aren't as easy anymore. These may include cooking, getting dressed, or just moving around. Some people can't work because of the pain or have to cut back on their hours. They may worry about money. Limits on work and everyday life may also make people less social, wanting to see others less often.

Research shows that people in pain may feel sad or anxious and may get depressed more often. At other times they may feel angry and frustrated. And they can feel lonely, even if they have others around them.

A common result of having cancer and being in pain is fear. For many, pain and fear together feel like suffering. People get upset worrying about the future.

They focus their thoughts on things that may or may not happen. You may feel fear about many things, such as fear of:

- The cancer getting worse
- The pain being too much to handle
- Your job or daily tasks becoming too hard to do
- Not being able to attend special trips or events
- Loss of control

This rollercoaster of feelings often makes people look for the meaning that cancer and pain have in their life. Some question why this could happen to them. They wonder what they did to deserve it. Others may turn to religion or explore their spirituality more, asking for guidance and strength.

Don't Lose Hope

If you have feelings like these, know that you're not alone. Many people with cancer pain have had these kinds of feelings. Having negative thoughts is normal. And some people have positive thoughts, too, finding benefits in facing cancer. But if your negative thoughts overwhelm you, don't ignore your feelings. Help is there for you if you're distressed or unsure about your future.

Finding Support

There are many people who can help you. You can talk with oncology social workers, health psychologists, or other mental health experts at your hospital or clinic. Your health care team can help you find a counselor who is trained to help people with long-term illnesses. These people can help you talk about what you are going through and find answers to your concerns. They may suggest medicine that will help you feel better if you need it.

Many people say that they regain a sense of control and well-being after talking with people in their spiritual or religious community. A leader from one of these groups may be able to offer support, too. Many are trained to help people cope with illness. Also, many hospitals have a staff chaplain who can counsel people of all faiths.

You can also talk with friends or others in your community. Some join a support group. Cancer support groups are made up of people who share their feelings about coping with cancer. They can meet in person, by phone, or over the Internet. They may help you gain new insights and ideas on how to cope. To find a support group for you, talk with your doctor, nurse, or oncology social worker.

How Your Pain Affects Your Loved Ones

Chronic or severe pain affects everyone who loves and takes care of you. It can be hard for family members and friends to watch someone close to them be in pain.

Like you, your loved ones may feel angry, anxious, and lonely. They may feel helpless because they can't make you feel better. They may even feel guilty that you have pain while they don't. Or they may feel loss, because your pain keeps you from doing things you like to do.

It's natural for family members and friends to have these emotions. It may help if everyone understands that these emotions exist and that no one needs to face them alone.

Let your family members know it's okay for them to get help. Like you, they can talk to a counselor or join a support group. Encourage them to ask the oncology social worker about the options that are available for them.

Also, they can read the NCI booklets for caregivers listed on the inside front cover of this booklet.

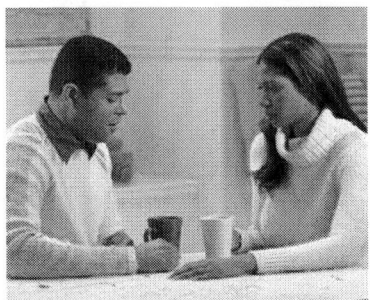

"I can't help feeling frustrated with all that's going on in my life. Between my cancer treatments and the pain, I get upset and angry. Sometimes I really need someone to talk to—someone who understands what I'm going through." —Carlos

Talking with Family Members

You may want to let family members and friends know how you're feeling. For some, this can be hard or awkward. Some people say that they want to avoid upsetting those closest to them. Others say that they don't want to seem negative. But open and honest communication can help everyone. Letting others know about your pain may help them understand what you are going through. They can then look for ways to help you. Your loved ones may also feel better knowing that they're helping to make you feel more comfortable.

Family Problems before Your Cancer

Any problems your family had before you got cancer are likely to be more intense now. Or maybe your family just doesn't communicate very well. If this is the case, you can ask a social worker to set up a family meeting for you. During these meetings, the doctor can explain treatment goals and issues. And you and your family members can state your wishes for care. These meetings can also give everyone a chance to express their feelings in the open. Remember, there are many people you can turn to at this time.

Chapter 9

Financial Issues

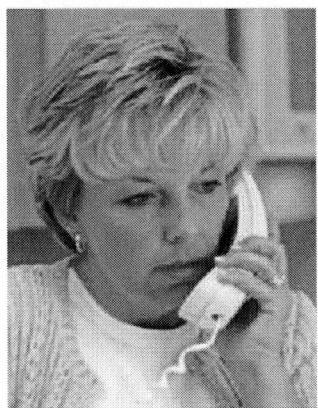

"My doctor told me about a pain control technique that he thought would help me. I was a little worried about how I would pay for it. It took one phone call to my insurance company, and my questions were answered." —Terry

When you're in pain, the last thing you want to think about is paying for your medicine. Yet money worries have stopped many people from getting the pain treatment they need. Talk with your oncology social worker if you have questions. He or she should be able to direct you to resources in your area. Here are some general tips:

Insurance

When dealing with health insurance, you might want to:

- Call your insurance company and find out what treatments are covered. Sometimes insurance companies pay for only certain types of medicines. If the medicine you need isn't covered, your doctor may need to write a special appeal letter. Or your doctor may need to prescribe a different treatment.
- Ask if your insurance company can give you a case manager to help you with your coverage.
- Check to make sure that your plan will cover any specialists your doctor refers you to. If it does not, check with your insurance company to see which doctors are included in your plan. Ask your doctor to refer you to someone on your plan's list.
- Find out whether you have to pay copayments up front and how much they cost.
- Find out how you should pay your balance. For example, do you file a claim? Does the insurance company pay first? Or do you pay and get reimbursed?
- Tell the insurance company if you believe you've received an incorrect bill. You should also tell your doctor or the hospital or clinic that sent the bill. Don't be afraid to ask questions.

Government Health Insurance

Medicare

Medicare is health insurance for people age 65 or older. However, people under 65 who are on kidney dialysis or have certain disabilities may also qualify.

Medicare Part B only pays for outpatient medicine given by a pump or by vein. It doesn't pay for pills, patches, or liquids.

Medicare Part D is a benefit that covers outpatient prescription medicines. It comes from private insurance plans that have a contract with Medicare. These plans vary in what they cost and the medicines they cover. Find out which medicines a plan covers before you join to make sure that it meets your needs. You should also know how much your copays and **deductible** will be.

Medicaid

Medicaid gives health benefits to low income people and their families. Some may have no health insurance or not enough, and therefore need this help.

If you have Medicaid, you should know that it pays for medicine given by mouth (**orally**) or by vein (intravenous). Each state has its own rules about who is eligible for Medicaid.

> To learn more about Medicare and Medicaid talk with your oncology social worker. You can also go to the Medicare and Medicaid Web site, **www.cms.hhs.gov**, or call the helpline at 1-800-MEDICARE (1-800-633-4227). Specialists can answer your questions or direct you to free counseling in your area.

Other Advice

Don't be embarrassed to tell your health care team if you're having trouble paying for your medicine. They may be able to prescribe other medicine that better fits your budget.

If you feel that you're overwhelmed, the stress may seem like too much to handle. You might try getting help with financial planning. Talk with the business office where you get treatment. There are many free consumer credit counseling agencies and groups. Talk with your oncology social worker about your choices.

You can also contact the NCI's Cancer Information Service (CIS) and ask for the **Financial Assistance and Other Resources for People With Cancer** fact sheet. See the Resources section on page 34 for ways to contact NCI.

Tips for Saving Money on Pain Medicine

If the cost of pain medicine is an issue for you, consider the following tips:

- Ask your doctor if there are **generic** brands of your medicine available. These usually cost less than brand-name medicines.
- Ask your doctor for medicine samples before paying for a prescription. You can't get samples of opioids. But you can ask your doctor to write only part of the prescription. This way you can make sure that the medicine

works for you before buying the rest of it. This will only help if you pay by the amount you buy. For some insurance plans, you pay the same amount for part of or the whole prescription. Find out what will work best for you.

Ask about drug companies that have special programs to give free drugs to patients in financial need. Your doctor should know about these programs.

Remember that pills may cost less than other forms of medicine.

Use a bulk-order mail pharmacy. But first make sure that the medicine works for you. Also, be aware that you can't order opioids in bulk or through the mail. Ask your oncology social worker or pharmacist about bulk-order mail pharmacies.

Contact NeedyMeds. They are a nonprofit organization that helps people who cannot afford medicine or health care costs. Go to www.needymeds.com or ask someone to do it for you.

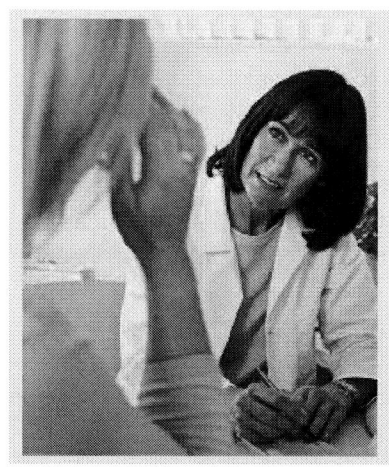

When the world says, "Give up," Hope whispers, "Try it one more time." (author unknown)

Reflection

You can take control of your pain. Work with your doctor and the other members of your health care team to find the best plan for you. Read the tips in this booklet and make them work for you. Don't lose hope. You don't have to accept pain as a normal part of cancer or treatment. You deserve to have the best care and support there is.

Resources

You can get information about cancer from many sources. Some are listed here. You may also want to check for more information from support groups in your community.

For More Resources

Go to the NCI web site at www.cancer.gov. In the search box, type in the words "national organizations. Or call 1-800-4-CANCER (1-800-422-6237) to seek more help.

Federal Agencies

- National Cancer Institute
  Has current information on cancer prevention, screening, diagnosis, treatment, genetics, and supportive care. NCI's web site (www.cancer.gov) lists clinical trials and specific cancer topics in NCI's Physician Data Query (PDQ®) database.

- Cancer Information Service
  Gives clear, up-to-date information on cancer to patients, families, health professionals, and the general public. It translates the latest scientific information into plain language in English, in Spanish, or on TTY equipment.

Toll-free: 1-800-4-CANCER (1-800-422-6237)
TTY: 1-800-332-8615
Online: www.cancer.gov/cis
Chat online: www.cancer.gov/help

- Centers for Medicare & Medicaid Services (CMS)
  Has information about patient rights, prescription drugs, and health insuranceissues, including Medicare and Medicaid.
  Toll-free: 1-800-MEDICARE (1-800-633-4227)
  Online: www.medicare.gov (for Medicare information) or www.cms.hhs.gov (for other information)

- National Center for Complementary and Alternative Medicine (NCCAM)
  Part of the National Institutes of Health. It funds and studies medical practices that are not commonly used as standard care. It rates how well these different practices work and shares this information with the public.
  Toll-free: 1-888-644-6226
  TTY: 1-888-644-6226
  Online: nccam.nih.gov

Private/Nonprofit Organizations

- American Cancer Society (ACS)
  Mission is to end cancer as a major health problem through prevention, saving lives, and relieving suffering. ACS works toward these goals through research, education, advocacy, and service. The organization's National Cancer Information Center answers questions 24 hours a day, 7 days a week.
  Toll-free: 1-800-ACS-2345 (1-800-227-2345)
  TTY: 1-866-228-4327
  Online: www.cancer.org

- American Pain Foundation
  Serves people with pain through information, advocacy, and support; pain and resource information, practical help and publications are available through toll-free telephone service and website.
  Toll-free: 1-888-615-PAIN (1-888-615-7246)

Resources

Online: www.painfoundation.org

- Cancer*Care*
  Offers free support, information, and financial and practical help to people withcancer and their loved ones.
  Toll-free: 1-800-813-HOPE (1-800-813-4673)
  Online: www.cancercare.org

- Center to Advance Palliative Care
  Goal is to increase the availability of quality palliative care services for people facing serious illness. Offers training and assistance to health care professionals.
  Phone: 1-212-201-2670
  Online: www.capc.org
  For patients: www.getpalliativecare.org and families:

- National Coalition for Cancer Survivorship (NCCS)
  Gives out information on cancer support, employment, financial and legal issues,advocacy, and related issues.
  Toll-free: 1-877-NCCS-YES (1-877-622-7937)
  Online: www.canceradvocacy.org

- National Hospice and Palliative Care Organization (NHPCO)
  Has information on hospice care, local hospice programs, advance directives in different states, and finding a local health care provider. It offers education and materials on palliative and end-of-life issues through its Caring Connections program, as well as links to other organizations and resources.
  Toll-free: 1-800-658-8898
  Online: www.nhpco.org
  Caring Connections
  Toll-free: 1-800-658-8898
  Online: www.caringinfo.org

- NeedyMeds
  Lists medicine assistance programs available from drug companies.
  NOTE: Usually patients cannot apply directly to these programs. Ask your doctor, nurse, or social worker to contact them.

Online: www.needymeds.com

- Patient Advocate Foundation
  Offers education, legal counseling, and referrals concerning managed care, insurance, financial issues, job discrimination, and debt crisis matters.
  Toll-free: 1-800-532-5274
  Online: www.patientadvocate.org

- The Wellness Community
  Provides free psychological and emotional support to cancer patients and their families.
  Toll-free: 1-888-793-WELL (1-888-793-9355)
  Online: www.thewellnesscommunity.org

Pain Control Record

You can use a chart like this to keep a record of how well your medicine is working. Some people call it a pain diary. Write the information in the chart below. Describe the amount of pain you feel using the way that works best for you. You can use words, numbers on a scale from 0 to 10, or even draw a face. Take the chart with you when you visit your doctor.

Date	Time	Describe the pain you feel	Level of pain
6/8 **(example)**	8 a.m.	stabbing pain in side	9
6/10 **(example)**	all day	dull ache in legs	5

Medicines You are Taking Now

Use this form to record all medicines—not just pain medicines—that you are taking. This information will help your doctor keep track of all your medicines.

Date	Medicine	Dose	How often taken	How well is it working?	Prescribing doctor

Pain Medicines You Have Taken in the Past

Use this form to record the pain medicines you have taken in the past. It will help your doctor understand what has and hasn't worked.

Date	Medicine	Dose	How often taken	Side effects	Reason for stopping

How to Use Imagery

Imagery usually works best with your eyes closed. To begin, create an image in your mind. For example, you may want to think of a place or activity that made you happy in the past. Explore this place or activity. Notice how calm you feel.

If you have severe pain, you may imagine yourself as a person without pain. In your image, cut the wires that send pain signals from one part of your body to another. Or you may want to imagine a ball of healing energy. Others have found this exercise to be very helpful:

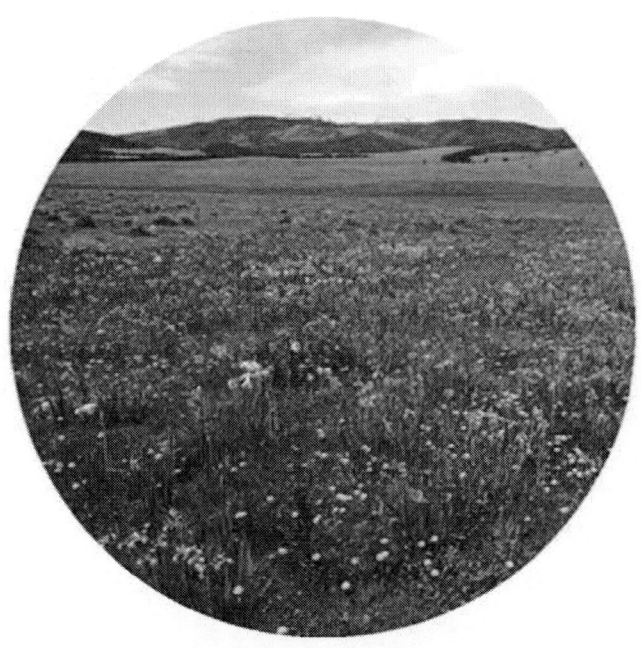

- Close your eyes and breathe slowly. As you breathe in, say silently and slowly to yourself, "In, one, two," and as you breathe out, say "Out, one, two." Do this for a few minutes.
- Imagine a ball of healing energy forming in your lungs or on your chest. Imagine it forming and taking shape.
- When you're ready, imagine that the air you breathe in blows this ball of energy to the area where you feel pain. Once there, the ball heals and relaxes you. You may imagine that the ball gets bigger and bigger as it takes away more of your discomfort.
- When you breathe out, imagine the air blowing the ball away from your body. As it goes, all your pain goes with it.
- Repeat the last two steps each time you breathe in and out.
- To end the imagery, count slowly to three, breathe in deeply, open your eyes, and say silently to yourself, "I feel alert and relaxed."

Relaxation Exercises

You may relax either sitting up or lying down, preferably in a quiet place. Make sure you're comfortable. Don't cross your arms or legs because you could cut off circulation. If you're lying down, you may want to put a small pillow under your neck and knees.

Once you're comfortable and your eyes are closed, you could try any of the following relaxation methods:

Breathing and Muscle Tensing

- Breathe in deeply.
- At the same time, tense your muscles or group of muscles. For example, you can squeeze your eyes shut, frown, or clench your teeth. Or, you could make a fist, stiffen your arms and legs, or draw your legs and arms up into a ball and hold as tightly as you can.
- Hold your breath and keep your muscles tense for a second or two.
- Let go. Breathe out and let your body go limp.

Slow Rhythmic Breathing

- Stare at an object or shut your eyes and think of a peaceful scene. Take a slow, deep breath.
- As you breathe in, tense your muscles. As you breathe out, relax your muscles and feel the tension leaving.
- Remain relaxed and begin breathing slowly and comfortably, taking about nine or 12 breaths a minute. To maintain a slow, even rhythm, you can silently say to yourself, "in, one, two; out, one, two."
- If you ever feel out of breath, take a deep breath, and continue the slow breathing.
- Each time you breathe out, feel yourself relaxing and going limp. Continue the slow, rhythmic breathing for up to 10 minutes, if you need it.
- To end the session, count silently and slowly from one to three. Open your eyes. Say to yourself, "I feel alert and relaxed." Begin moving slowly.

If you decide to use slow rhythmic breathing as a way to relax and reduce pain, you may want to try these tips. They can add to the experience.

- Listen to slow, familiar music through earphones.
- Once you're breathing slowly, slowly relax different parts of your body, one after the other. Start with your feet and work up to your head.
- Each time you breathe out, you can focus on a particular area of the body and feel it relaxing. Try to imagine the tension draining from the area.
- Consider using relaxation tapes. They often include each step on how to relax.

Words to Know

Acupuncture (ACK-yu-punk-chur): Small needles are inserted into the skin at certain points of the body to relieve pain. Acute pain: Pain that is very bad but lasts a fairly short time. Addiction (uh-DIK-shin): Drug craving, seeking, and use that you can't control.

Analgesic: A drug that reduces pain. Anesthesiologist (an-uh-steez-ee-YAH-luh-jist): A doctor who specializes in giving medicines or other drugs that prevent or relieve pain.

Anticonvulsant (an-tee-kuhn-VUHL-sint): Medicine used to treat seizures that can also be used to control burning, stabbing, and tingling pain. Antidepressant (an-tee-duh-PRES-int): Medicine used to treat depression that can also be used to relieve tingling, stabbing, or burning pain from damaged nerves.

Biofeedback: A way of learning to control some body functions such as heartbeat, blood pressure, and muscle tension with the help of special machines. This method may help control pain.

Breakthrough pain: An intense rise in pain that occurs suddenly or is felt for a short time. It can occur by itself or in relation to a certain activity. It may happen several times a day, even when you're taking the right dose of medicine.

Chemotherapy (kee-moh-THAIR-uh-pee): Treatment with anticancer medicines.

Chronic (KRAH-nik) pain: Pain that can range from mild to severe and is present for a long time.

Complementary treatment: Treatment used along with standard medical care. Deductible: The amount you must pay for health care before insurance begins to pay.

Distraction: A pain relief method that takes the attention away from the pain.

Dose: The amount of medicine taken.

Epidural (ep-uh-DUR-ul): An injection into the spinal column but outside of the spinal cord. Having to do with the space between the wall of the spinal canal and the covering of the spinal cord.

Generic: The scientific name of a drug, as opposed to the brand name. Also, drugsnot protected by trademark.

Hypnosis (hip-NOH-sis): A person enters into a trance-like state, becomes more aware and focused, and is more open to suggestion.Imagery: People think of pleasant images or scenes, such as waves hitting a beach,to help them relax.

Integrative medicine: Combines standard medical care and complementary and alternative medicine, for which there is some high-quality evidence of safety and effectiveness.

Intravenous (in-tra-VEE-nus): Within a blood vessel. Also called **IV**.

Intravenous infusion: A way of giving pain medicine into a vein or under the skin. An infusion flows in by gravity or a mechanical pump. It is different from aninjection, which is pushed in by a syringe.

Laxative: Something you take to help you pass solid waste, or stool, from your body. There are many different kinds of laxatives.

Narcotics (nahr-KAH-tiks): See opioids.

Nerve block: Pain medicine is injected directly into or around a nerve or into the spine to block pain.

Neurologist: A doctor who specializes in the treatment of nervous system disorders.

Neuropathic (noor-AH-path-ik) **pain:** Pain that occurs when treatment damages the nerves.

Nonopioids (nahn-OH-pee-yoidz): Acetaminophen and nonsteroidal anti-inflammatory drugs (NSAIDs), such as aspirin, ibuprofen, and naproxen.

Nonprescription: Over-the-counter drugs that you can buy without a doctor's order.

NSAIDs (Nonsteroidal anti-inflammatory drugs): Medicines that control mild to moderate pain and inflammation and reduce fever. Can be used either alone ortogether with other medicines.

Oncologist (ahn-KAH-luh-jist): A doctor who specializes in the treatment of cancer.

Oncology (ahn-KAH-luh-jee): The study and treatment of cancer.

Onset of action: The length of time it takes for a medicine to start to work.

Opioids (OH-pee-yoidz): Also known as narcotics. They are used to treat moderateto severe pain. A prescription is needed for these medicines.

Oral: By mouth. Pain threshold: The point at which a person becomes aware of pain.
Palliative (PAL-ee-yuh-tiv) **care:** Care given to improve quality of life and/or slow cancer's growth. The goal is to prevent or treat the symptoms, side effects, and psychological and emotional problems of the disease. Not meant to be a cure.
Patient-controlled analgesia (an-ull-JEEZ-ya) **(PCA):** A way for a person with pain to control the amount of pain medicine he or she receives. When pain relief is needed, the person can press a button on a computerized pump connected to a small tube inserted into the vein or under the skin. Pushing the button delivers a preset dose of pain medicine.
Phantom pain: When pain or other unpleasant feelings are felt from a missing (phantom) body part that has been removed by surgery.
Physical therapy: Treatment for pain in muscles, nerves, joints, and bones. Thistreatment uses exercise, electrical stimulation, and hydrotherapy, as well as massage,heat, cold, and electrical devices.
Prescription: A doctor's order.
Qi (chee)**:** What is believed to be a life force energy.
Radiation therapy: Treatment with high-energy x-rays to kill or control cancer cells.
Relaxation techniques: Methods used to lessen tension, reduce anxiety, andmanage pain.
Side effects: Problems caused by a medicine or other treatment. Examples are constipation and drowsiness.
Skin patch: A bandage-like patch that releases medicine through the skin and theninto the bloodstream. The medicine enters the blood slowly and steadily.
Standard treatment: The treatment that is accepted and most often used.
Stage: The extent of disease. It can also be a phase of a clinical trial.
Steroids: Medicines that reduces swelling and inflammation.
Stool softeners: Medicine that softens the solid waste in your body, making it easier to pass.
Subcutaneous (sub-kyu-TAY-nee-yus) **injection:** A shot under the skin.
Sublingual: Under the tongue.
Supplements: Vitamins, minerals, herbs, and other things you can take besides medicines.
Tolerance: Occurs when the body gets used to a medicine. The result is that the dose no longer works well. Either more medicine is needed to control the pain ordifferent medicine is needed.

Transcutaneous (tranz-kyu-TAY-nee-yus) **Electrical Nerve Stimulation (TENS):** A method in which mild electric currents are applied to some areas of theskin by a small power pack connected to two electrodes.

Transmucosal (tranz-myu-KO-sol)**:** Absorbed through the lining of the mouth.

Withdrawal: Signs and symptoms that can appear when long-term use of opioidsis stopped or suddenly reduced a lot.

Important Names and Phone Numbers

Doctor _____

Doctor _____

Nurse _____

Clinic _____

Pharmacist _____

Other _____

Appointments

_____

_____

_____

Before You go to the Pharmacy—Know What You're Getting!

Sometimes people get new prescriptions and are confused about how to take them and when. If your doctor prescribes a new medicine, it's important for you to understand what you will be taking.

Before you leave your visit, ask your health care team:

- How do you spell the name of the drug?
- What does the medicine look like? If there is a generic version, does it look the same?
- How many pills (or how much liquid) are in *each* dose?
- How many *times a day* do I take the dose?
- Should I take this medicine with food?
- Can I take it with my other medicine or supplements?

Be sure to read the printed information that comes with your medicine. If you have trouble reading it, ask a friend or family member to read it for you.

Index

A

acetaminophen, 20, 22
acupuncture, 37, 38, 42
addiction, 33, 34, 35
advocacy, 54, 55
age, 48
alcohol, 21, 25, 28
allergic reaction, 17
alternative, 10, 64
alternative medicine, 64
anticancer drug, 21
anti-inflammatory drugs, 20, 64
anxiety, viii, 37, 40, 41, 65
appetite, 2
arthritis, 22
ash, 63
availability, 55
awareness, 39

B

baths, 39
beer, 21, 28
beliefs, 13
biofeedback, 37, 38
biopsy, 6
bladder, 7
bleeding, 20, 21, 22
blocks, 29
blood, 20, 22, 40, 63, 64, 65
blood flow, 40
blood pressure, 63
bloodstream, 65
bone marrow, 6
bone marrow test, 6
bowel, 7, 24
brain, 29
breathing, 17, 25, 38, 39, 41, 42, 61
burning, 6, 10, 26, 63

C

cancer, iv, vii, viii, 1, 2, 5, 6, 9, 15, 16, 19, 23, 25, 26, 27, 33, 34, 35, 37, 38, 40, 41, 42, 43, 44, 45, 46, 51, 53, 54, 55, 56, 64, 65
cancer cells, 65
caregivers, 45
chee, 65
chemotherapy, 20, 22
Chinese medicine, 37
circulation, 39, 60
CIS, 49
clinical trials, 53
communication, 10, 46
community, 44, 45, 53
concentration, 41, 42
Congress, iv
constipation, 23, 24, 65

control, iv, vii, viii, 1, 2, 9, 10, 11, 15, 16, 17, 19, 20, 23, 24, 25, 26, 33, 34, 35, 37, 38, 44, 47, 51, 63, 64, 65
cooking, 43
cough, 20
coughing, 7
counsel, 44
counseling, 49, 56
covering, 27, 64
craving, viii, 33, 63
credit, 49
cultural beliefs, 13

D

database, 53
debt, 56
Department of Health and Human Services, 12
depression, 3, 26, 40, 63
diarrhea, 26
directives, 55
discomfort, 6, 37, 60
discrimination, 56
dizziness, 17
doctors, vii, 2, 7, 9, 11, 23, 27, 29, 48
drug addict, 33
drugs, vii, 10, 16, 19, 20, 22, 25, 26, 30, 50, 54, 63, 64

E

elderly, 21
electric current, 30, 66
electrodes, 66
emotions, 41, 45
employment, 55
energy, 29, 37, 41, 42, 59, 60, 65
exercise, 40, 41, 59, 65

F

family, 2, 10, 13, 16, 45, 46, 69

family members, 45, 46
fatigue, 40
fear, 43
fears, 9
feedback, vii, 9
feelings, viii, 40, 43, 44, 45, 46, 65
feet, 61
fever, 19, 20, 21, 64
financial planning, 49
focusing, 40
food, 24, 28, 69
fruits, 24
funds, 54

G

gel, 39
genetics, 53
glasses, 24
goals, 46, 54
gout, 22
gravity, 64
groups, vii, 2, 19, 44, 45, 49, 53
growth, 65
guidance, 44
guilty, 45

H

hands, 40
harm, viii, 33
healing, 59, 60
health, vii, viii, 1, 5, 9, 10, 11, 13, 15, 16, 17, 23, 25, 26, 37, 38, 44, 48, 49, 50, 51, 53, 54, 55, 63, 69
health care, vii, viii, 1, 9, 10, 11, 13, 15, 16, 17, 23, 25, 26, 37, 38, 44, 49, 50, 51, 55, 63, 69
health care costs, 50
health care professionals, 55
health insurance, 48, 49, 54
health problems, 10
heart disease, 21
heart rate, 38

heartburn, 20
heat, 39, 65
heating, 39
hip, 64
hospice, 55
hospitals, 38, 44
hypnosis, 37, 39, 42

I

ibuprofen, 20, 21, 22, 64
imagery, 37, 40, 41, 60
images, 39, 64
income, 49
infection, 20
inflammation, 20, 21, 64, 65
injections, 27
injury, iv
insurance, 47, 48, 50, 56, 63
intimacy, 2

J

joints, 65

K

kidney, 21, 22, 48
kidney dialysis, 48
knees, 60

L

language, 53
laxatives, 24, 64
learning, 38, 63
legal issues, 55
links, 55
liquids, 24, 27, 48
listening, 38
liver, 20, 21
liver damage, 21
lying, 60

M

machinery, 28
Medicaid, 49, 54
medical care, 63, 64
Medicare, 48, 49, 54
mental health, 44
messages, 1, 29
milk, 20
mind-body, 40, 42
money, viii, 9, 43, 47
morning, 39
motion, 40
movement, 24, 41
muscle strain, vii, 5
muscles, 39, 41, 60, 61, 65
music, 38, 41, 61

N

narcotics, 22, 64
National Institutes of Health, 54
nausea, 19, 25, 38
nerve, 26, 29, 64
nervous system, 42, 64
New York, iv
NSAIDs, 20, 21, 22, 64
nurses, vii, 2

O

older people, 20
opioids, vii, 19, 22, 23, 24, 25, 26, 34, 49, 50, 64

P

pain, iv, vii, viii, 1, 2, 5, 6, 7, 9, 10, 11, 13, 15, 16, 17, 19, 20, 21, 22, 23, 24, 25, 26, 27, 28, 29, 30, 33, 34, 35, 37, 38, 39, 40, 41, 42, 43, 44, 45, 46, 47, 49, 51, 54, 57, 58, 59, 60, 61, 63, 64, 65
pain management, 33

palliative, 2, 17, 55
patient rights, 54
PCA, 27, 65
physical therapy, 42
planning, 22
poor, 39
power, 30, 66
pressure, 37, 40
prevention, 53, 54
program, 55
psychiatrist, 39
psychologist, 39
pumps, 27

Q

quality of life, viii, 37, 65

R

radiation, 6, 26, 29, 65
radiation therapy, 6
range, vii, 5, 63
reading, 39, 69
rectum, 20, 27
relaxation, 41, 60, 61
religion, 44
resources, viii, 47, 55
rhythm, 61
routines, 2

S

safety, 64
saving lives, 54
search, 53
sensation, 37, 39
shape, 60
shares, 54
shortness of breath, 41
side effects, viii, 2, 11, 19, 20, 23, 26, 29, 65
sign, 6
signals, 59

skin, 24, 27, 37, 63, 64, 65
sleeping pills, 25
social workers, 2, 44
solid waste, 64, 65
spinal cord, 6, 27, 64
spine, 6, 29, 64
spirituality, 44
stomach, 20, 21, 22, 23
stomach ulcer, 22
strength, 41, 44
stress, viii, 37, 40, 41, 49
subcutaneous injection, 27
supply, 39
sweat, 26
swelling, 19, 21, 26, 65
symptoms, 2, 20, 25, 26, 65, 66

T

technician, 38
teeth, 60
telephone, 54
television, 38
temperature, 21
tension, 38, 40, 41, 61, 63, 65
therapy, 29, 41, 65
threshold, 10, 65
tin, 26, 37, 63
training, 55
tranquilizers, 25
trial, 65
tumor, 6, 29, 30

V

vegetables, 24
vein, 27, 48, 49, 64, 65
vomiting, 24, 38

W

walking, 24, 25
web, 42, 53

wires, 59
withdrawal, 26
worry, viii, 9, 33, 34, 40, 43

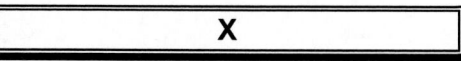

x-rays, 65